so,

you

have

cancer...

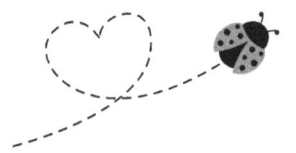

christina repetti

so, you have cancer . . .

ISBN: 979-8-9920547-0-5 Paperback
ISBN: 979-8-9920547-1-2 Hardcover
ISBN: 979-8-9920547-2-9 eBook

Printed in the United States

Editor: Kevin Anderson & Associates
Cover Design and Interior Formatting: Becky's Graphic Design®, LLC

Royalty Free Artwork Purchased from Adobe Stock Library

Dedicated to my Mom and Dad.

Mom, you never missed a doctor's appointment. You did everything to try to make me feel better and more comfortable, with endless love and support.

Dad, you always kept the sun shining, even on rainy days, and reminded me the rain will eventually stop falling after this storm.

The both of you had enough strength for the entire family. I love you so much!!!

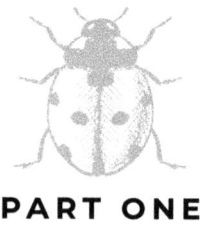

PART ONE

the good

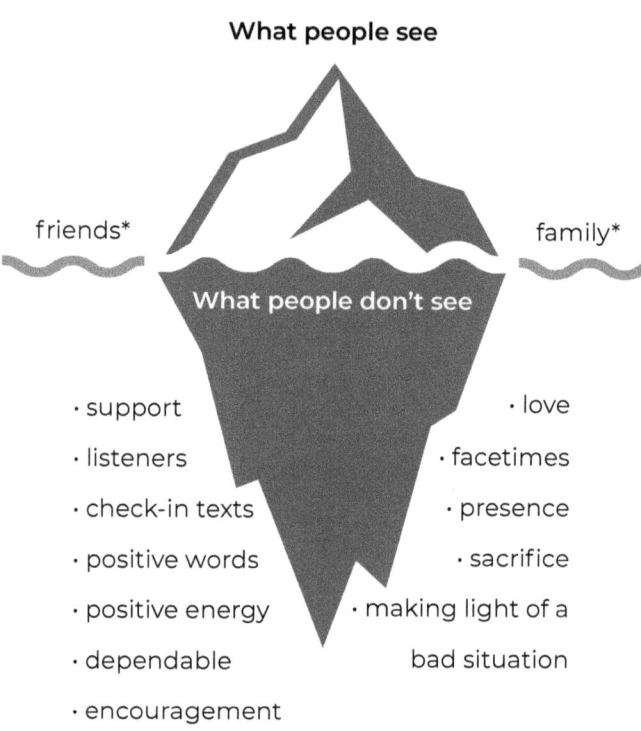

What people see

friends*

family*

What people don't see

- support
- listeners
- check-in texts
- positive words
- positive energy
- dependable
- encouragement

- love
- facetimes
- presence
- sacrifice
- making light of a
  bad situation

On my window, on my arm.

At the beach, a ladybug

my lucky charm.

Follow me from place to place

showing me everything will be okay.

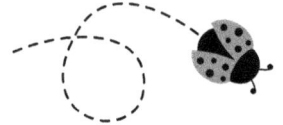

You're dealt a certain hand in life.

It is what it is.

Take the deal, and run with it.

You can't change what's happened, but you can determine how you react to it.

And sometimes, that's enough to sway the outcome in your favor.

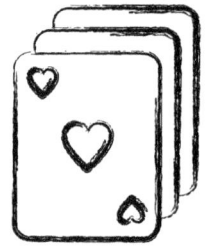

When life gives you cancer, you meet cancerAIDES 🧑‍⚕️

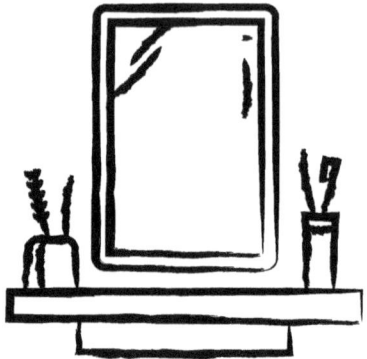

I am suddenly 23. In the mirror, I see what is left of my hair. What is left of me. 70% gone. I try to lift it up. I try to lift me up. 70% gone. I'm scared to lose it all. But is it time for it to go?

I am 23.

In a few days, Dad will shave it off. He will remind me I will grow more.

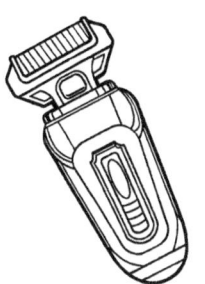

The razor started going.

Nerves creeped in.

Relief was near.

With each chunk of hair hitting the floor, my smile grew wider.

I could relax now, it's all gone.

I'm free.

Hi bb just wanna let you know I'm thinking about you and sending you a lot of love <3

How are you doing?

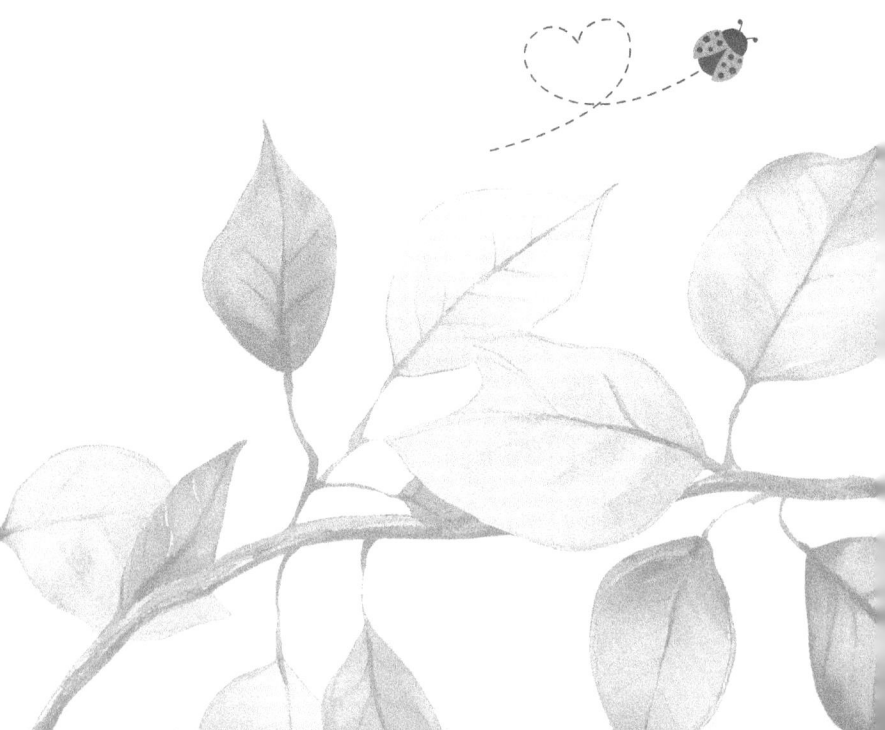

The breeze on my naked head feels so good.

I rub sunscreen on it.

My head now feels as smooth as butter.

Who would've thought I'd actually enjoy
some things about being bald???

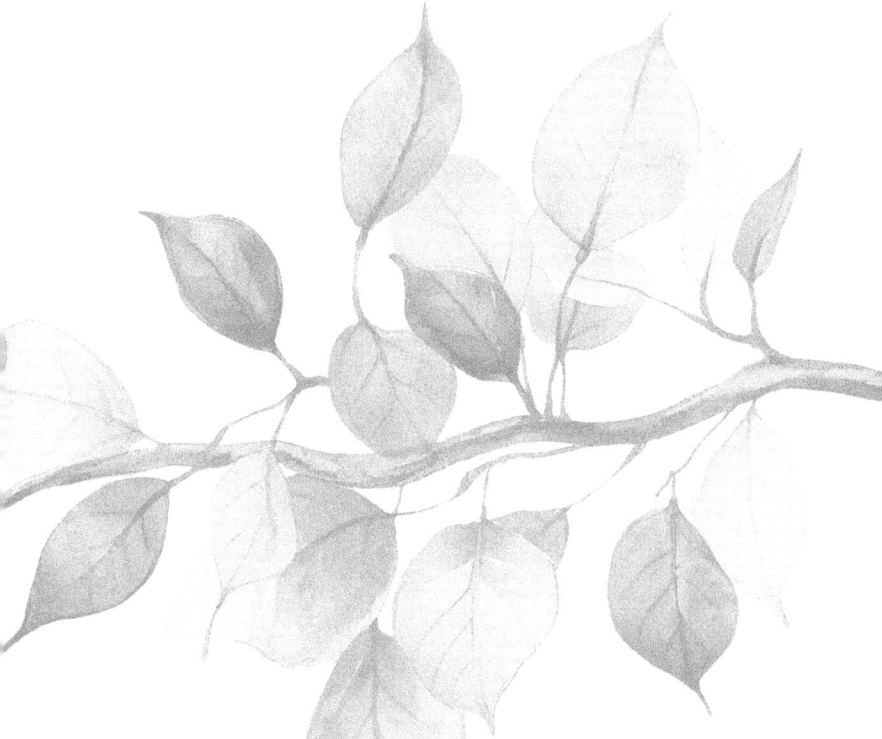

strength.
courage. brav-
ery. positivity.
love. family.
friends. believer. bal-
ance. bold. calm. cheery.
comfort. cooperative. de-
termined. emotional. faith-
ful. fearless. grateful. help-
ful. kindness. living. lucky.
queen. reassurance. resil-
ient. sharing. shimmer-
ing. support. thank-
ful. vivacious.

A close friend of mine takes a sip of my drink: "Wait, is cancer contagious?"

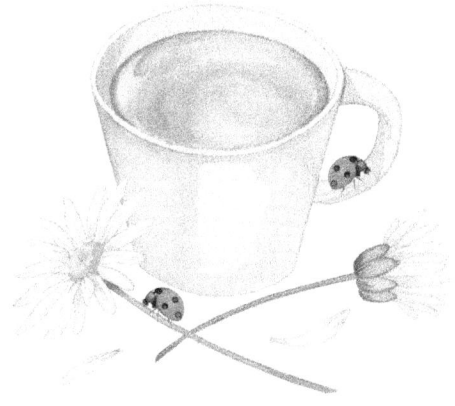

The needle goes deep into my spinal cord.

I can feel

Migraines

For days.

No sitting up

Straight.

Aches on aches on aches.

Check-ins,

FaceTimes and visits too,

Made the bad times

Not so blue.

Family, friends,

Friends of friends and nurses too,

make the blue a lighter hue.

Fighting isn't easy. Staying positive isn't easy. Eating isn't easy. Getting out of bed isn't easy. Showering isn't easy. Using the bathroom isn't easy. Smiling isn't easy. But, seeing my loved ones see me like this . . . is love.

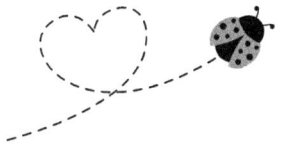

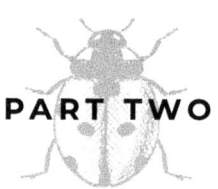

PART TWO

the bad

Most days go like this:

wake up.

take pills.

drink water.

eat toast.

take a nap.

wake up.

drink water.

eat a rice cake.

drink more water.

watch tv.

take pills.

sleep.

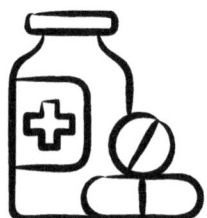

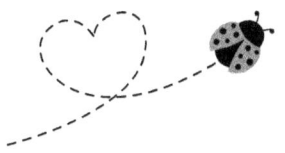

We sat there with cascading tears.

And heart-pounding fears.

Tears, fears, and bad news. What to do?

Everything is unknown. I have cancer.

What next?

How are you doing? Your hair will grow back! I completely understand being scared and upset about that but you will always be BEAUTIFUL. I'm so sorry you have to go through this, you are truly one of the most amazing people in my life and I wish it wasn't you who had to suffer through this. I love you so much.

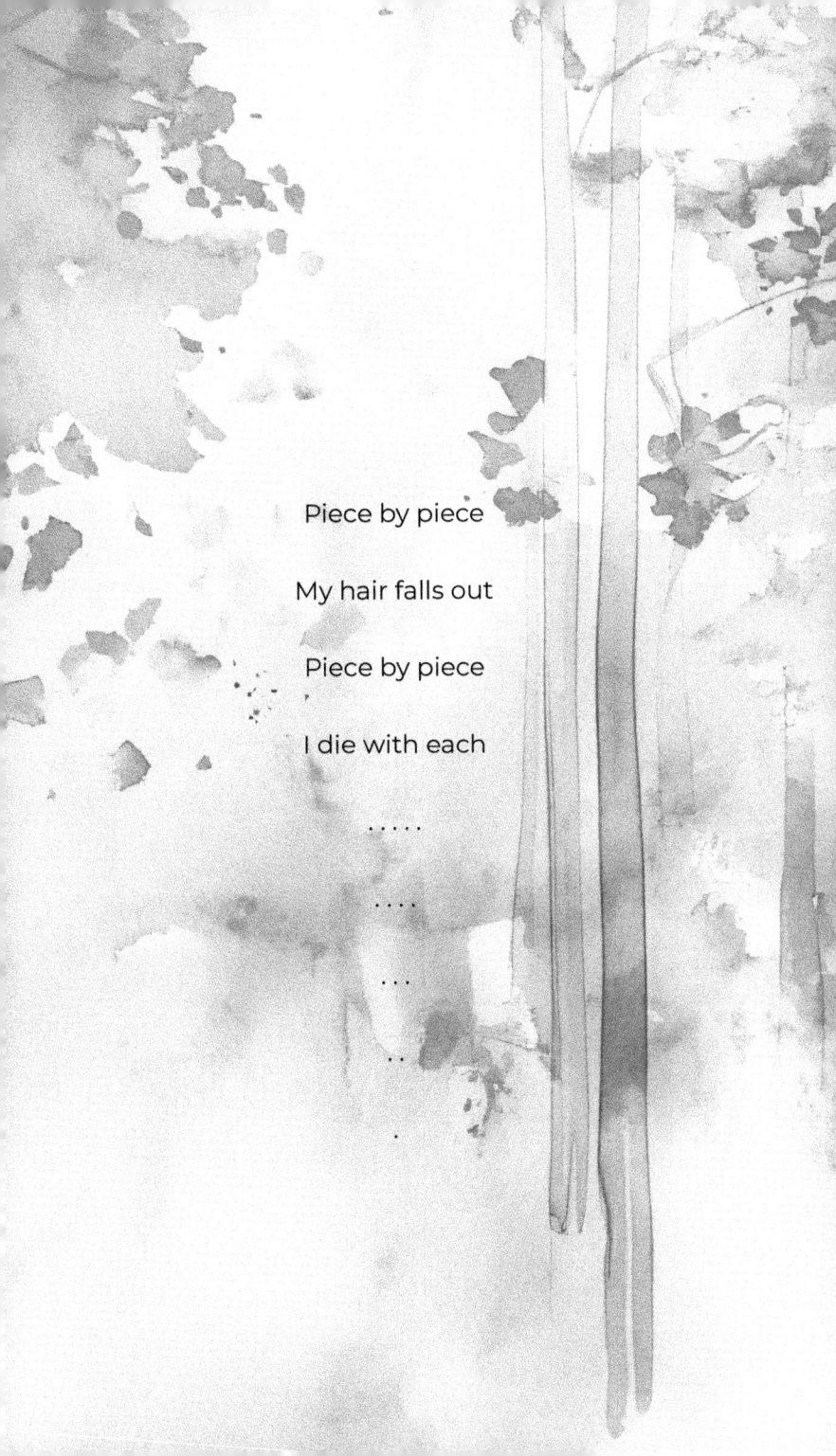

Piece by piece

My hair falls out

Piece by piece

I die with each

. . . . .

. . . .

. . .

. .

.

You're gonna be the nurses favorite patient

you know it!!

Is this a fucking dream?

A nightmare. Am I breaking down?

My hair clumps. A nightmare.

I run my fingers through my hair.

It falls out. The chemo kicked in.

In the car, on my pillow, on the back of my shirt.

A nightmare. I can't brush it, I can't wash it

I can't touch it, it hurts. A nightmare.

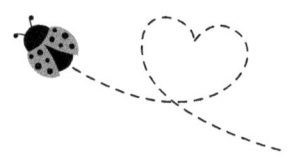

Your chances are less than 1%, they said.

Sounds pretty rare.

But, we already knew that about me.

No one knew a beast was growing inside me.

It grew and grew until it ripped open my insides.

When are they getting you a bed?

If you want, I can go down there and throw someone out of a bed!

lol. Hopefully soon

I'm bedridden

And moving too fast makes everything go black.

Getting up hurts. Loud sounds make my headache worse.

I eat breakfast in bed, drink water, and sleep.

My bed is the only place I find comfort.

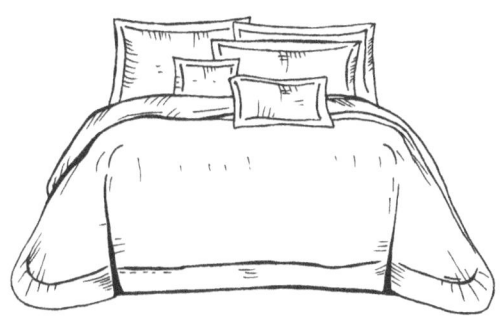

A poke here, a stick there. All I see is 1%.

I know you would rather not go through this nor would any of us want you to go through it, but it's obviously a necessity now.

It will be fine.

Everything will work out for the best.

I have cancer. It's hard to hear
& even harder to say.

I have cancer. . .

It's 2 am and my face is plunging toward the toilet bowl.

This is a first.

I heave and then breathe, heave then breathe.

Sending my love and reiki healing to you. You're not in this alone kiddo. Love you lots!!!! 🙏🤍

They say "beauty is pain."

They weren't lying.

Bare

Excruciating

Ache

Uncovered

Tragedy

Yucky

Bald is beautiful.

Beep . . . beep . . . beep . . . beep.

On repeat, I'm hooked up

To get a poisonous treat.

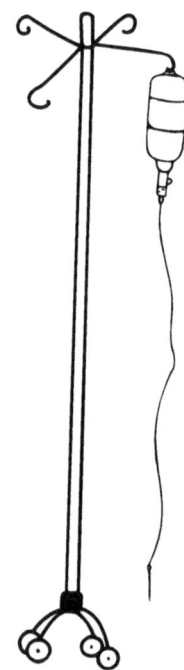

Yesterday is gone. Tomorrow has not yet come. We have only today. Let us begin.

JOSEPH CARDINAL BERNARDIN

Good luck. My family is keeping you in our thoughts 🙏🏻🙏🏻

YOU WILL BEAT THIS

KNOCKIN' ON HEAVEN'S DOOR

Kn- kn- knockin' on the spinal cord.

Mama put my pills on the table.

I can't take them anymore.

That cold, sharp needle is
coming down.

Feels like they're knockin' on the
spinal cord.

Kn-kn- knockin' on the spinal cord.

Kn-kn- knockin' on the spinal cord.

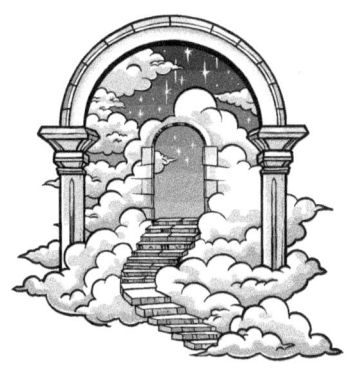

1 water

2 waters

3 waters

4

a few more waters and you won't hit
the floor!

Chug chug chug!!!

Shotgun a water lol

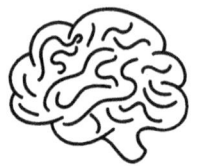

Chemo brain is real. Forgetting what you ate for breakfast. Forgetting conversations with friends. Forgetting if you took your pills. Be patient. Your memory will return soon enough.

Do not fear for I am with you. Do not be afraid for I am your God. I will strengthen you, I will help you, I will uphold you...

Isaiah 41:10

Each bad day is one day closer to freedom.

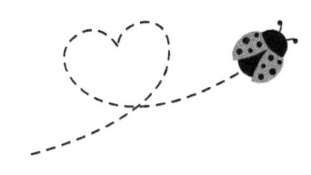

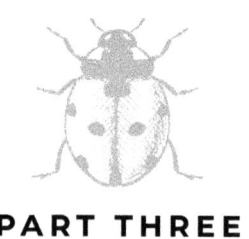

PART THREE

The can-you-
believe-it's-
a-happy-
ending

Hospital stays:

Visitors &

talking,

tv &

phone,

uno &

crosswords,

bloodwork &

chemo.

Finally,

all done.

I wish I could take the pain from the sick faces I see along the way.

It feels weird to be happy for myself, knowing that I'll be okay.

You're a fighter and I have your back every step of the way.

Let's kick some cancer butt.

You can and
you will!

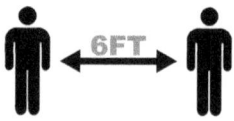

Visits from friends & family.

Six feet.

No hugs.

But I still feel complete.

My brain tells me to seem lively.

Don't forget to laugh and let those lips curl.

Take another bite of my food.

Just to prove I'm in the mood.

I'm holding my stomach tightly.

About to hurl.

Hold it in.

Breathe.

How untimely.

15 stairs.

You can do it.

5 down.

Take a break.

Hold the railing,

Up you go.

Now catch a breath.

Made it.

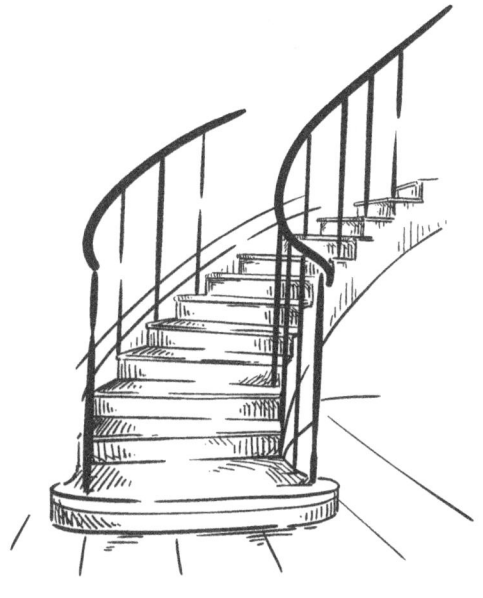

I know your last treatment is coming up, wanted to say good luck and I'm praying for you. Kick its ass 🙏 🩶

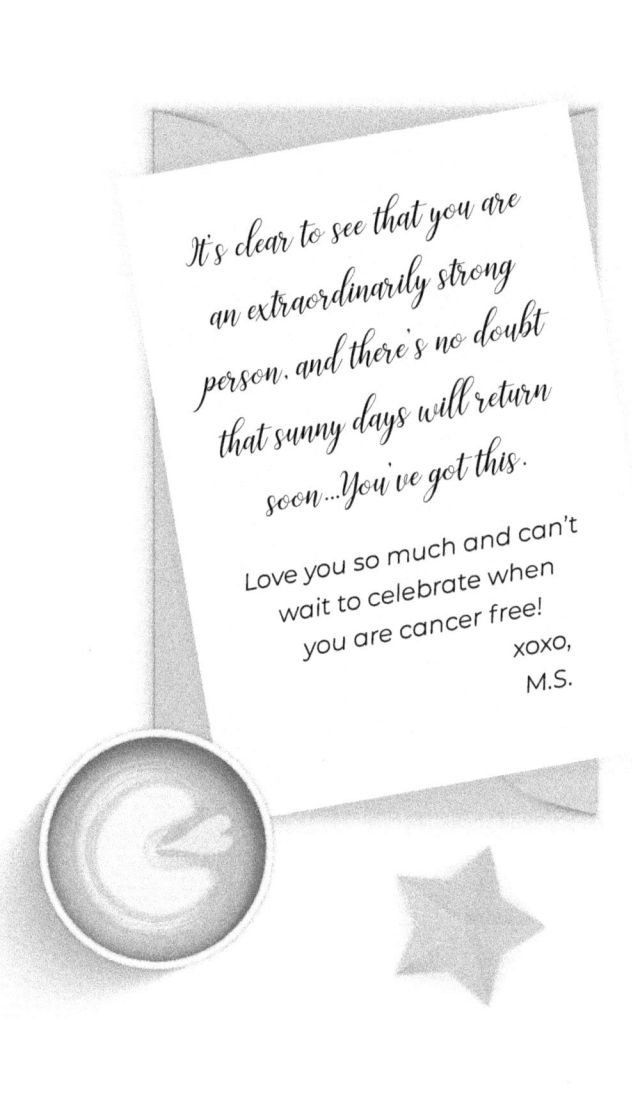

It's clear to see that you are an extraordinarily strong person, and there's no doubt that sunny days will return soon...You've got this.

Love you so much and can't wait to celebrate when you are cancer free!

xoxo,
M.S.

The peach fuzz is growing.

It's so soft on my head and light like sand.

Every day it grows and each month

I feel more whole.

Ladybug wings wrapped around me.

Protection from harm.

Protection from hurt.

Protecting me so that God wouldn't take me too soon.

Now, I have ladybug wings branded on me in honor of the protection they gave me.

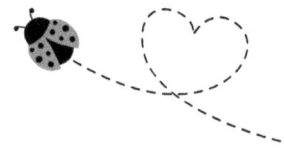

Comparisons I've gotten through my hair growth stages:

- Demi Moore (G.I Jane)
- Justin Timberlake
- Princess Diana
- Little Annie
- Shirley Temple
- Molly Ringwald
- Farrah Fawcett
- Rosie the Riveter
- Marilyn Monroe

Compliments here, compliments there. Everyone thinks I should keep my hair. Why grow it longer they say? Short is a slayyyy!

Why me? I asked.

Because you can beat it, cancer answered.

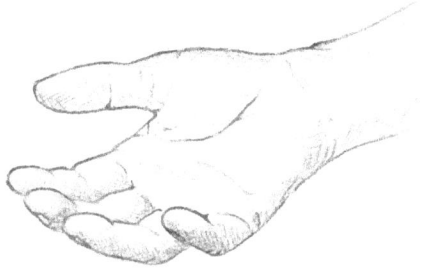

Protect me God, for I have shown you strength and positivity through the bad times behind me now. I've proved I'm worthy. Only good lies ahead here on out.

July 29th:

I put my middle finger up and said
goodbye to cancer. I'm finally free.

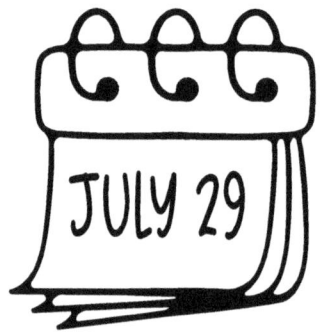

Ring the bell!!!!

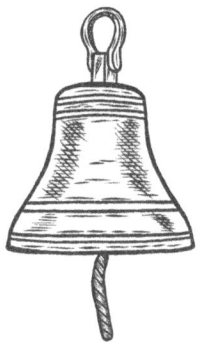

GLADLY!!!!

God chose me.

I have yet to figure out why.

But one day, it'll hit me. The reason why will have already come & passed by then.

It will be an afterthought.

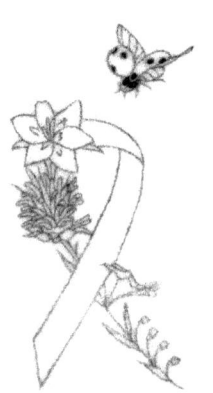

about the author

It all began when I was in extreme abdominal pain one night that landed me in the ER the next morning. After hours of waiting, the doctors concluded that I had appendicitis. They performed surgery to find that my appendix had burst and I would be there for a few more days. They sent my appendix out for testing as it had an abnormal shape to it, besides being twice the size of a normal appendix.

The doctors said there was a less than 1% chance that it could have a tumor. I thought my odds were pretty good. I was very wrong. At my follow-up appointment, I was told I had Non-Hodgkin's Lymphoma. The unfortunate journey to then follow, led me to a beautiful realization. I am made for more.

There is more purpose for me on this earth.

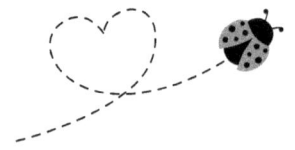

acknowledgments

For all my angels up above who saved me. This book,
nor I, wouldn't be here without you.